NCLEX: Pharmacology for Nurses

105 Nursing Practice Questions & Rationales to EASILY Crush the NCLEX!

Chase Hassen

Nurse Superhero

© 2015

Disclaimer:

Although the author and publisher have made every effort to ensure that the information in this book was correct at press time, the author and publisher do not assume and hereby disclaim any liability to any party for any loss, damage, or disruption caused by errors or omissions, whether such errors or omissions result from negligence, accident, or any other cause.

This book is not intended as a substitute for the medical advice of physicians. The reader should regularly consult a physician in matters relating to his/her health and particularly with respect to any symptoms that may require diagnosis or medical attention.

NCLEX®, NCLEX®-RN, and NCLEX®-PN are registered trademarks of the National Council of State Boards of Nursing, Inc. They hold no affiliation with this product.

Have you seen my other NCLEX Prep Books?
NCLEX: Respiratory System : 105 Nursing Practice Questions and Rationales to Easily Crush the NCLEX!

NCLEX: Endocrine System : 105 Nursing Practice Questions and Rationales to EASILY Crush the NCLEX!

NCLEX: Cardiovascular System : 105 Nursing Practice and Rationales to Easily Crush the NCLEX!

NCLEX: Emergency Nursing : 105 Practice Questions and Rationales to Easily Crush the NCLEX!

EKG Interpretation: 24 Hours or Less to Easily Pass the ECG Portion of the NCLEX!

Lab Values: 137 Values You Know to Easily Pass The NCLEX!

First, I want to give you this FREE gift...

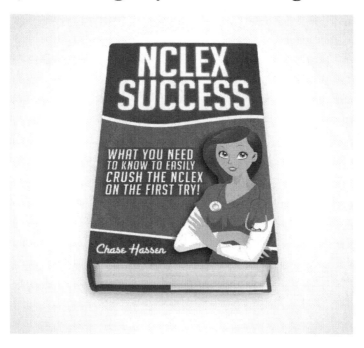

Just to say thanks for downloading my book, I wanted to give you another resource to help you absolutely crush the NCLEX Exam.

For a limited time you can download this book for FREE.

http://bit.ly/1VNGAZ9

Table of Contents

Chapter 1 : NCLEX: Pharmacology Questions

The following are 105 questions that will help you study for the NCLEX evaluation. All of the questions are based on things you might need to know in the area of pharmacology. Following the quiz will be the identical questions with the answers and rationales. Compare your answers with the correct ones to see where you may need to study some more. Good luck!

PLEASE NOTE: The answers are located in the next chapter. If you would prefer to see the questions and answers as you review this study guide, visit page 57.

1. The nurse is giving insulin to a client with diabetes for what purpose?
   a. To relieve disease manifestations
   b. For preventative reasons
   c. For health maintenance
   d. For curative purposes

Answer:

2. In asking for a medication history, which questions will elicit the most accurate information?
   a. "Do you take any herbal supplements?"
   b. "What time of day do you go to bed?"
   c. "What is the highest level of education you completed?"
   d. "Do you have vision or hearing impairment?"
   e. "Where do you eat most of your meals?"
   f. "Do you have drug insurance coverage?"

Answer:

3. Which should the nurse include in the oral drug administration procedure?
   a. Administer a drug to a three year old as a capsule.
   b. Administer two drugs at a time to an older adult client.
   c. Administer a carbonated beverage over ice after giving a drug.
   d. Administer a sustained release buccal drug under the tongue.

Answer:

4. Which should the nurse do when administering drugs by nasogastric tube?
   a. Crush the drug before administering through a feeding tube.
   b. Flush between drugs with 10 cc of sterile water.
   c. Give one drug with 30 cc of water.
   d. Keep the client upright for fifteen minutes after giving the drug.

Answer:

5. What is a priority for the nurse to consider before giving a parenteral injection to a two-year-old child?
   a. Apply EMLA and prilocaine to the site an hour before giving the injection.
   b. Lightly tap on the injection site before giving the injection.
   c. Give up to 1 cc of the drug to the injection site.
   d. Use the vastus lateralis for giving the drug.

Answer:

6. The nurse chooses which isotonic IV solution for hydration, while being able to give potassium as well?
   a. 0.45% NaCl solution
   b. Dextrose 5 percent solution
   c. Dextrose in 0.45% solution
   d. Ringer's lactate

Answer:

7. The nurse gives a heparin injection with a tuberculin syringe that has what volume?

Answer:_____

8. The nurse gives Demerol IM to an adult by choosing which sized needle?
   a. 16 gauge
   b. 18 gauge
   c. 23 gauge
   d. 26 gauge

Answer:

9. The nurse is giving a unit of packed RBCs. Which should the nurse look for if the client is having an acute hemolytic reaction? Select all that apply.
   a. Tachycardia
   b. Headache
   c. Fever
   d. Hypertension
   e. Dyspnea
   f. Back pain

Answer:

10. The nurse should use what gauge of needle to administer blood?

Answer: _____

11. When giving IV therapy to a client, it would be necessary for the nurse to include which of the following aspects of the procedure?
    a. Make a time strip on the bag with a felt tip marker.
    b. Change the tubing every 24 hours.
    c. Replace the IV solution with the same solution when the current bag runs out.
    d. Avoid letting an IV bag hang more than 24 hours

Answer:

12. The nurse should include the following when administering an IV solution?
    a. Choose a microdrip chamber for medications given to a child.
    b. Set the end time of an infusion pump to give off an alarm 20 minutes before the scheduled end time.
    c. Select a macrodrip chamber for medications given to a geriatric client.
    d. Choose a volume-controlled administration set to deliver a large amount of IV solution.

Answer:

13. The nurse hangs which of the following for a client with thrombocytopenia?
    a. Whole blood
    b. Packed RBCs
    c. Platelets
    d. Albumin

Answer:

14. A nurse cares for a client with a peripheral IV. Which would indicate the client is experiencing hypervolemia? Select all that apply.
    a. Nausea and vomiting
    b. Headache
    c. Dyspnea
    d. Hypertension
    e. Fever
    f. Tachycardia

Answer:

15. The nurse is caring for a client with an IV that is experiencing dyspnea, hypotension, a weak and rapid pulse, a decreased level of consciousness, and cyanosis. What is a priority nursing intervention?
    a. Notify the physician
    b. Place the client in a Trendelenburg position
    c. Give oxygen
    d. Stop the IV

Answer:

16. The client is receiving fresh frozen plasma. The nurse should follow what lab results to see if the therapy is working?
    a. Hemoglobin and hematocrit
    b. Platelets
    c. Prothrombin time and partial thromboplastin time
    d. White blood cells

Answer:

17. You are teaching a class on controlled substances. What should you include as part of the class?
    a. There is no accepted medical use for a Schedule I controlled substance.
    b. Examples of Schedule II drugs include glutethimide, secobarbital, and hydrocodone.
    c. Schedule III controlled substances have a high potential for abuse.
    d. Schedule IV controlled substances are the same as an over-the-counter medication.

Answer:

18. Guaifenesin belongs to what class of controlled substances?
    a. Schedule II
    b. Schedule III
    c. Schedule IV
    d. Schedule V

Answer:

19. The nurse is giving a client blood. Which of the following means that the nurse does not understand how to give blood?
    a. Run the blood slowly for the first 15 minutes at 20 drops per minute.
    b. Establish the required flow rate after 15 minutes if no signs of a reaction.
    c. Transfuse the blood slowly over six hours.
    d. Assess the vitals every 30 minutes until 1 hour after the transfusion.

Answer:

20. Which of the following clients is most appropriate to receive a central venous catheter?
    a. A dehydrated client with hypokalemia who needs fluid and electrolyte replacement.
    b. A client with cancer of the esophagus who is receiving chemotherapy.
    c. A client with an infection who needs short-term antibiotics.
    d. A client who is postoperative and is experiencing nausea after surgery.

Answer:

21. The nurse should question the use of which drug for use in a client with glaucoma?
    a. Diamox
    b. Pilocarpine
    c. Atropine Sulfate
    d. Mannitol

Answer:

22. The nurse is giving a beta blocker to a client with glaucoma. What would indicate that there is a serious adverse reaction?
    a. Photophobia
    b. Blurry vision
    c. Drop in blood pressure
    d. Worsening of asthma

Answer:

23. What does a nurse give to a client with keratitis?
    a. Acyclovir
    b. Diamox
    c. Scopolamine
    d. Stoxil

Answer:

24. The nurse is administering Timoptic in each eye. Which comment does the client say indicating the need for more teaching?
    a. "I must wash my hands before putting in the drops."
    b. "This drug will decrease the fluid in my eye."
    c. "I need to take this until my eye pressure is normal."
    d. "Adverse reactions include dizziness and double vision."

Answer:

25. The nurse tells client that the best position for instilling nose spray is to what?
    a. Bend the head forward
    b. Push the nare to the side
    c. Tilt the head backward
    d. Open the mouth to facilitate breathing

Answer:

26. You are assigned to give eyedrops to a client getting ready for cataract surgery. What kind of eye drop are you to give?
    a. An osmotic diuretic
    b. A miotic agent
    c. A mydriatic agent
    d. A thiazide diuretic

Answer:

27. The nurse is giving a topical anti-infective whenever she gives the following: Select all that apply.
    a. Amoxicillin
    b. Polymixin B
    c. Neomycin
    d. Ceclor
    e. Chloramphenicol
    f. Biaxin

Answer:

28. A client has Meniere's disease and asks why Antivert is being prescribed. How does the nurse respond?
    a. It will control the vertigo.
    b. It will help you sleep.
    c. It will decrease your pain.
    d. It will control your nausea.

Answer:

29. A client is receiving phenylephrine (Neo-Synephrine). What should the nurse monitor the client for? Select all that apply.
    a. Urinary retention
    b. Dry skin
    c. Hypertension
    d. Tachycardia
    e. Headache
    f. Decreased sensitivity to light

Answer:

30. The nurse is taking a medication history from a client with herpes simplex of the eye. The nurse should ask if the client is taking which of the following drugs?
    a. Viroptic
    b. Cromolyn
    c. Stoxil
    d. Diamox

Answer:

31. The nurse understands that a client is to get which of the following drugs to paralyze the ciliary body muscles?
    a. Phenylephrine
    b. Homatropine
    c. Paredrine
    d. Cromolyn

Answer:

32. A client has been receiving IV theophylline and the doctor discontinues the medication to begin an immediate-release form of the medication. When should the first dose of the oral medication be given?
    a. Right after stopping the IV theophylline
    b. Begin 4-6 hours after stopping the IV theophylline
    c. Begin the oral dose at bedtime
    d. Start the oral dose with morning medications

Answer:

33. The client with acute asthma has inspiratory and expiratory wheezing along with a decreased FEV. What class of prescribed drugs should be given first to the client?
    a. Oral steroids
    b. Bronchodilators
    c. Inhaled steroids
    d. Mucolytics

Answer:

34. The nurse is treating a client with asthma who is to be on theophylline. Which is an appropriate question to ask the client?
    a.   Are you a diabetic on insulin?
    b.   Do you take Tagamet?
    c.   Do you regularly take aspirin?
    d.   Do you exercise routinely?

Answer:

35. After teaching a client to use a beclomethasone inhaler, what does the client say to indicate that the teaching has been successful?
    a.   I will limit myself to 2 cups of coffee per day.
    b.   I will take it with meals to mask the taste.
    c.   I will take it before bedtime every night.
    d.   I will rinse my mouth after each use.

Answer:

36. The client is being instructed as to how to use cromolyn sodium. Which indicates the client needs further instruction?
    a. If I don't feel better in 2-3 weeks, I will stop taking the medication.
    b. I will call the doctor if I get severe coughing from the drug.
    c. I have to take the medication even when I feel good.
    d. I do not need to stop my other medications just because I am taking this one.

Answer:

37. The client is being instructed on how to use a metered dose inhaler. What should the nurse tell the patient to do?
    a. Hold the breath for three seconds after using the inhaler
    b. Take a quick breath when activating the canister
    c. Activate the canister at the beginning of a slow deep breath
    d. Place the canister six inches in front of an open mouth

Answer:

38. What are the appropriate inhalation drugs for inflammation? Select all that apply.
    a. Cortisone
    b. Beclomethasone
    c. Dexamethasone
    d. Flunisolide (Aero-Bid)
    e. Prednisone
    f. Azmacort

Answer:

39. The client with asthma asks why corticosteroids are best given by inhalation. What do you say?
    a. Inhaled medications are easier to take.
    b. The systemic adverse reactions are reduced.
    c. No weaning is required when stopping the drug.
    d. Oral care is not required.

Answer:

40. The client has a sudden asthma attack. Which inhaler should the nurse give first?
    a. Albuterol
    b. Azmacort
    c. Flovent
    d. Cromolyn

Answer:

41. A client has pneumonia and is on a ventilator for respiratory distress. The chest x-ray shows left lower lob consolidation. The doctor orders respiratory treatments with Mucomyst. The nurse should monitor the client for what effects of the treatment?
    a. Bronchodilation
    b. Increased sputum
    c. Decreased level of consciousness
    d. Hypotension

Answer:

42. The nurse is caring for a client with an intractable cough. Which drug should be administered to the client?
   a. Rifampin
   b. Mucomyst
   c. Flovent
   d. Codeine

Answer:

43. What should the nurse give as a priority to a client with a positive TB skin test but no evidence of active disease?
   a. Repeat skin test in 6 months.
   b. Isoniazid for 12 months.
   c. Multidrug therapy for at least 12 months.
   d. Streptomycin for 12 months.

Answer:

44. The nurse is giving a client isoniazid. How should the medication be given to absorb the best?
    a. On an empty stomach
    b. With antacids to relieve upset stomach
    c. With food
    d. Thirty minutes after meals.

Answer:

45. You are caring for a client with COPD and pneumonia. After removing the endotracheal tube, which order should be in question?
    a. Continuation of antibiotics.
    b. O2 per nasal cannula at 6 liters/minute
    c. Out of bed with assistance
    d. Continue nebulizer treatments

Answer:

46. Humidification is necessary for oxygen flow rates of greater than what for drying of the mucus membranes?
    a. 1 liter/min
    b. 2 liter/min
    c. 3 liter/min
    d. 4 liter/min

Answer:

47. You are teaching a client on the appropriate use of nebulizers and metered dose inhalers. What should you include as part of your instructions?
    a. Metered dose inhalers require a gas flow rate of 6-10 liters/min
    b. Nebulizers give medication through a face mask or mouthpiece
    c. Nebulizers deliver medications in puffs
    d. Metered dose inhalers need to be refrigerated

Answer:

48. Which of the following are adverse drug reactions for bronchodilators? Select all that apply.
    a. Headache
    b. Tachycardia
    c. Sneezing
    d. Back pain
    e. Palpitations
    f. Depression

Answer:

49. You are delegating nursing tasks. What task should you designate to the LPN?
    a. Monitor the client using a decongestant for drug effectiveness.
    b. Develop a teaching plan for effective coughing techniques for a client on an expectorant.
    c. Increase the O2 flow rate for a client receiving O2 by face mask.
    d. Give a nasal spray to a client with rhinitis.

Answer:

50. A client is in status asthmaticus. What is a priority nursing action?
    a. Administer aminophylline IV per doctor's order.
    b. Monitor the respiratory status for signs of hypoxia.
    c. Give inhaled bronchodilator therapy as ordered.
    d. Provide emotional support.

Answer:

51. Which of the following is a priority activity for a nurse to do before administering digoxin?
    a. Assess the apical pulse for one minute.
    b. Palpate the radial pulse for 60 seconds.
    c. Monitor renal function tests.
    d. Assess the serum potassium.

Answer:

52. A client is in cardiac arrest. Which drug should the nurse give first?
    a. Atropine
    b. Epinephrine
    c. Lidocaine
    d. Atenolol

Answer:

53. After teaching a client about atenolol, which indicates the diabetic client understands the instructions given?
    a. It may cause hyperglycemia.
    b. It may mask an early indication of hypoglycemia.
    c. It may increase the action of insulin.
    d. It may lessen the effectiveness of insulin.

Answer:

54. The nurse is taking care of a client with hypertension. Which drug should be administered?
    a. Mexiletine
    b. Dyazide
    c. Digoxin
    d. Warfarin

Answer:

55. The client is receiving nitroglycerin for angina. What is the action of nitroglycerin on the body?
    a. Increase afterload
    b. Increase preload
    c. Constrict the arteries
    d. Dilate the veins

Answer:

56. The nurse is caring for a client with atrial fibrillation. Which drug concentration will double if given with quinidine?
    a. Lasix
    b. Digoxin
    c. Propranolol
    d. Dyazide

Answer:

57. The nurse is giving amiodarone in order to treat which kind of arrhythmia?
    a. Sinus bradycardia
    b. Bundle branch block
    c. Ventricular arrhythmia
    d. Junctional rhythm

Answer:

58. Which is a priority nursing intervention for a client receiving adenosine for SVT?
    a. Document the presence of peripheral pulses.
    b. Monitor the pulse oximetry
    c. Assure the IV is in the antecubital vein.
    d. Prepare for emergency defibrillation.

Answer:

59. A client on Viagra is also experiencing angina for which the doctor has prescribed nitroglycerin as needed. What should the nurse tell the client about the taking of these two medications?
    a. Viagra should not be used within 24 hours of taking nitroglycerin.
    b. Nitroglycerin and Viagra should be taken at the same time.
    c. Viagra is not effective when used with nitroglycerin.
    d. The effect of nitroglycerin is impaired when used with Viagra.

Answer:

60. Which adverse reaction should the nurse assess in an elderly client receiving a continuous infusion of lidocaine?
    a. Hypertension
    b. Osteoarthritis
    c. Confusion
    d. Decreased visual acuity

Answer:

61. The nurse is giving a beta blocker for unstable angina because it has which of the following actions?
    a. It increases myocardial contractility
    b. It decreases heart rate
    c. To promote a cardiovascular fluid shift
    d. For coronary artery vasodilation

Answer:

62. What is a priority nursing action when giving a client an ACE inhibitor?
    a. Monitor the blood pressure closely for 2 hours after the first dose.
    b. Begin with a high dose and then taper down the dose.
    c. Give potassium supplements to the client.
    d. Begin with daily dosing followed by every other day dosing.

Answer:

63. The nurse is instructing a client on the use of Plavix. Which client statement indicates an understanding of the use of the drug?
    a. "I should ambulate slowly."
    b. "I may experience hypotension."
    c. "I should use caution taking other drugs that cause bleeding."
    d. "I should take a stool softener while on this drug."

Answer:

64. The nurse should monitor a client with a heart attack that is receiving IV streptokinase for what serious adverse reaction?
    a. Intracranial hemorrhage
    b. Intractable nausea
    c. Extension of myocardial infarction
    d. Pulmonary embolism

Answer:

65. The nurse is caring for a client on Lipitor. The client drinks 6-12 beers per day. What should the nurse look out for as a potentially serious adverse reaction to the drug?
    a. Nephrotoxicity
    b. Hypertension
    c. Hepatotoxicity
    d. Dyspepsia

Answer:

66. The client understands that the Zantac he is taking does what?
    a. Decreases gastric acid levels
    b. Changes hormonal levels.
    c. Increases pepsin levels
    d. Decreases pH levels.

Answer:

67. Which of the following should the nurse tell the client who is taking Carafate?
    a. It reduces gastric acid production
    b. It is to be given at breakfast time.
    c. Separate the taking of Carafate with other drugs by 2 hours.
    d. Carafate acts against H. pylori.

Answer:

68. Which is a priority drug to give to a client who has gastroesophageal reflux disease (GERD)?
    a. Cytoprotectors
    b. Antibiotics
    c. Proton pump inhibitors
    d. Anticholinergics

Answer:

69. The nurse should assess which of the following body systems while giving IV Tagamet to the client?
    a. Urinary system
    b. Immune system
    c. Respiratory system
    d. Cardiovascular system

Answer:

70. The nurse should monitor the client taking Prevacid for which adverse reactions? Select all that apply.
    a. Headache
    b. Oliguria
    c. Anxiety
    d. Dry mouth
    e. Diarrhea
    f. Decreased appetite

Answer:

71. The client is experiencing peptic ulcer disease due to H. pylori. Which drug combinations should be given? Biaxin is given along with what?
    a. Tetracycline and sodium bicarbonate
    b. Flagyl and Amphogel
    c. Amoxicillin and Prilosec
    d. Penicillin and Axid

Answer:

72. The nurse tells the client that which antacid has the side effect of constipation?
    a. Magaldrate (Riopan)
    b. Maalox
    c. Aluminum carbonate (Basaljel)
    d. Milk of Magnesia

Answer:

73. The nurse is caring for a client with a 15 year history of gastric ulcers. What should be taken by the client for minor aches and pains?
    a. Acetaminophen
    b. Buffered aspirin
    c. Plain aspirin
    d. Ibuprofen

Answer:

74. Which of the following antacids should the nurse question giving to the client with gastric ulcer and CHF?
    a. Magaldrate (Riopan)
    b. TUMS
    c. Milk of Magnesia
    d. Sodium bicarbonate

Answer:

75. The nurse is providing a medication schedule for a client taking Mylanta for gastritis. To promote best absorption, this drug should be given when? Select all that apply.
    a. At bedtime
    b. 1 hour before meals
    c. Immediately after meals
    d. Upon arising in the morning
    e. 1 hour after meals
    f. Thirty minutes after meals

Answer:

76. A client giving a medication history tells you she is in the early stages of pregnancy. Which drug should be immediately discontinued?
    a. Misoprostol (Cytotec)
    b. Docusate
    c. Magnesium Hydroxide
    d. Pepto-Bismol

Answer:

77. The nurse is giving a client Tagamet. Which of the following adverse reactions should be watched out for? Select all that apply.
    a. Tinnitus
    b. Alopecia
    c. Diarrhea
    d. Mental confusion
    e. Dizziness
    f. Dyspepsia

Answer:

78. The nurse chooses the best antacid for the client because of which characteristic?
    a. Sweet-tasting, cathartic and effective for a long period of time.
    b. Short acting and readily absorbed
    c. Not absorbed by the body and acts as a laxative
    d. Decreases acidity without constipation or diarrhea.

Answer:

79. After giving Actigall with a client who has gallbladder disease, the nurse expects the priority outcome to be what?
    a. Decreased vomiting
    b. Increased comfort
    c. Decreased stone formation
    d. Decreased bile production

Answer:

80. The nurse has given Compazine several times to a client experiencing vomiting. Which adverse reactions should the nurse be looking out for?
    a. Bradycardia
    b. Weight loss
    c. Akathisia
    d. Orthostatic hypotension
    e. Acute dystonia
    f. Oliguria

Answer:

81. The client is receiving somatropin (Humatrope). What should the nurse tell the client to do?
    a. Get an annual bone age assessment.
    b. Schedule a fasting blood sugar annually if there is a family history of diabetes mellitus.
    c. Record height weekly and report linear growth of 7-15 cm in the first year.
    d. Notify the physician if the urine output increases.

Answer:

82. Which of the following is an anticipated outcome for a client with diabetes insipidus receiving vasopressin injections?
    a. Urine output of 2500 cc/day
    b. Weight loss of 4 pounds in a week.
    c. Urine specific gravity of 1.005
    d. Oral intake of 4500 cc/day

Answer:

83. The client on vasopressin asks why they should avoid alcohol while on this medication. What do you say?
    a. Alcohol will increase vasoconstriction.
    b. Alcohol will decrease the antidiuretic effect.
    c. Alcohol will interfere with the absorption of vasopressin in the stomach.
    d. Alcohol will promote a hypersensitivity to vasopressin.

Answer:

84. The nurse recognizes that one of the following drugs is a first generation sulfonylurea in the treatment of diabetes? Select all that apply.
   a. Glipizide (Glucotrol)
   b. Tolbutamide (Orinase)
   c. Acarbose (Precose)
   d. Tolazamide (Tolinase)
   e. Chlorpropamide (Diabenese)
   f. Rosiglitazone (Avandia)

Answer:

85. Before discharge, the nurse instructs a patient on Cytomel to notify the physician if which of the following occurs?
   a. A pulse rate of 100 beats per minute.
   b. A weight loss of 5 pounds in two weeks.
   c. More frequent urination
   d. Excessive sleepiness

Answer:

86. The best time to take Synthroid (levothyroxine) is when?
    a. One hour after a meal.
    b. With a bedtime snack.
    c. Thirty minutes before breakfast.
    d. Once a day with any meal.

Answer:

87. The nurse is giving the client Mestinon. The client should be monitored for which of the following adverse reactions?
    a. Constipation
    b. Decreased heart rate
    c. Hypertension
    d. Increased intraocular pressure.

Answer:

88. The nurse should monitor the client for which signs after giving Ativan IV to a client who has many seizures?
    a. Tachycardia
    b. Hypertension
    c. Tissue hypoxia
    d. Respiratory depression

Answer:

89. A client is taking Dilantin 200 mg daily. Which of the following is an adverse reaction that must be watched out for?
    a. Diarrhea
    b. Pruritus
    c. Sedation
    d. Hypertension

Answer:

90. You are infusing Dilantin with which of the following solutions to control seizures?
    a. Normal saline
    b. D5W
    c. Lactated Ringer's solution
    d. D5W in 0.5 normal saline

Answer:

91. Dilantin is being given to a client for seizures. What should the nurse prepare to do?
    a. Maintain a level of between 30 and 50 micrograms per ml.
    b. Dilute the IV Dilantin with 5% dextrose
    c. Administer good oral hygiene.
    d. Give the medication intramuscularly.

Answer:

92. The nurse should tell a client taking an oral retinoid to
    avoid which of the following items?
    a. Dairy products
    b. Carbonated beverages
    c. Extremely cold air
    d. Vitamin A supplements

Answer:

93. The nurse is caring for a client who has been taking
    Accutane for the past two months. What is a priority
    condition that the nurse should report to the
    physician?
    a. Itching
    b. Depression
    c. Dry skin
    d. Headache

Answer:

94. The nurse is giving instructions to a client with itching to take an oral antihistamine to relieve itching. Which should be included in the instructions?
    a. The effects will be better if you take the medication around the clock.
    b. Take the medication only when the itching is at its worst.
    c. You can take the oral medication along with a topical antihistamine.
    d. Increase the dose of the oral antihistamine if the itching gets worse.

Answer:

95. A client has second-degree burns on the hands and arms. The client is being given Silvadene for topical antimicrobial effects. What instructions for taking the medication should be given?
    a. Wash the area with warm water before applying Silvadene.
    b. Apply a salve after the Silvadene to seal the medication into the burned area.
    c. Apply Silvadene using sterile technique
    d. Apply the medication only at bedtime.

Answer:

96. A 22-year old female has been diagnosed with acne
    and is starting on tetracycline. What is a priority
    question to ask the client before starting therapy?
    a. How long have you had acne?
    b. When was your last menstrual period?
    c. How many times a day do you wash your face?
    d. Have you been taking any oral medication for
       acne?

Answer:

97. The nurse tells the client that what is a good
    treatment for Raynaud's phenomenon?
    a. Nonsteroidal anti-inflammatory medication
    b. Corticosteroids
    c. Aspirin
    d. Calcium-channel blockers

Answer:

98. Allopurinol and colchicine have been prescribed for a client with gout and diabetes. How should you instruct the client?
    a. Tell them that blood glucose values may not be valid.
    b. Urine sugar tests may not be valid.
    c. Protein restrictions can lead to diabetic ketoacidosis.
    d. Protein cannot be restricted so you need to increase the dose of allopurinol.

Answer:

99. The nurse should give the following medications to a client with severe rheumatoid arthritis?
    a. Methotrexate
    b. Naproxen
    c. Aspirin
    d. Plaquenil

Answer:

100.   Which of the following should a nurse consider before giving an opioid to a child?
   a. The child's age, weight, height, and respiratory status.
   b. Children are less susceptible to adverse reactions.
   c. Addiction is increased in children.
   d. Sedation is increased in children.

Answer:

101.   When giving a child Augmentin, the nurse should monitor the client for what?
   a. Constipation
   b. Polyuria
   c. Decreased temperature
   d. Increased bleeding

Answer:

102.   The nurse is instructing a class about antibiotics and UTIs. Which should be included in the class?
   a. E. coli is mostly resistant to penicillin medications.
   b. Sulfonamides are given for Pseudomonas infections
   c. Fluoroquinolones have limited use in the treatment of UTIs.
   d. Cephalosporins are the treatment of choice for those sensitive to penicillin.

Answer:

103.   The nurse is admitting a client with suspected schizophrenia. Which of the following clinical manifestations should the nurse assess as a positive clinical manifestation of schizophrenia?
   a. Anhedonia and blunted affect.
   b. Hallucinations and delusional thinking
   c. Lack of motivation
   d. Abnormal movements of the mouth.

Answer:

104.   The nurse is caring for an Alzheimer's patient
who is taking Seroquel for paranoid ideations. Which
adverse reactions should the nurse look out for?
a. Hypertension
b. Headache
c. Bradycardia
d. Diarrhea
e. Dry mouth
f. Tardive dyskinesia

Answer:

105.   What should the nurse tell a client who is on an
antidepressant drug?
a. Drink low calorie beverages.
b. Instruct the client to take the drug on an empty
stomach.
c. Tell the client that urinary frequency is a side
effect of the drug.
d. The client should be monitored for bradycardia
before giving the drug.

Answer:

Great Job! On the next chapter, you will see the questions you
just answered plus the answers and rationales! I hope you did
well!

Chapter 2 : NCLEX: Pharmacology Questions, Answers, and Rationales

The following are the same questions you just took with the answers and rationales. Compare your answers with the correct answers to see where you may need to study further.

1. The nurse is giving insulin to a client with diabetes for what purpose?
    a. To relieve disease manifestations
    b. For preventative reasons
    c. For health maintenance
    d. For curative purposes

Answer: c. Insulin is used to control blood sugar, which is a part of health maintenance in a diabetic. It cannot prevent diabetes nor can it cure it. It does not change disease manifestations as there are no overt manifestations of disease in the daily life of a diabetic.

2. In asking for a medication history, which questions will elicit the most accurate information?
   a. "Do you take any herbal supplements?"
   b. "What time of day do you go to bed?"
   c. "What is the highest level of education you completed?"
   d. "Do you have vision or hearing impairment?"
   e. "Where do you eat most of your meals?"
   f. "Do you have drug insurance coverage?"

Answer: a. d. f. It is important to know if the client is taking herbal supplements and if they have problems reading the bottle or understanding drug recommendations. Insurance coverage is important because it affects their ability to pay for their medications.

3. Which should the nurse include in the oral drug administration procedure?
   a. Administer a drug to a three year old as a capsule.
   b. Administer two drugs at a time to an older adult client.
   c. Administer a carbonated beverage over ice after giving a drug.
   d. Administer a sustained release buccal drug under the tongue.

Answer: c. If you give a drug and then give a carbonated beverage over ice, it decreases the risk of nausea. Drugs should be given one at a time in the elderly and in liquid form in kids under 5. A buccal drug is given in the inside of the cheek.

4. Which should the nurse do when administering drugs by nasogastric tube?
   a. Crush the drug before administering through a feeding tube.
   b. Flush between drugs with 10 cc of sterile water.
   c. Give one drug with 30 cc of water.
   d. Keep the client upright for fifteen minutes after giving the drug.

Answer: c. Each drug should be given with 30 cc of water. Drugs shouldn't be given through a feeding tube because it is much too narrow. The client should be upright for 30 minutes after giving the drug.

5. What is a priority for the nurse to consider before giving a parenteral injection to a two-year-old child?
   a. Apply EMLA and prilocaine to the site an hour before giving the injection.
   b. Lightly tap on the injection site before giving the injection.
   c. Give up to 1 cc of the drug to the injection site.
   d. Use the vastus lateralis for giving the drug.

Answer: d. The priority item is the selection of the site. The other things are true but are not the priority over the site.

6. The nurse chooses which isotonic IV solution for hydration, while being able to give potassium as well?
   a. 0.45% NaCl solution
   b. Dextrose 5 percent solution
   c. Dextrose in 0.45% solution
   d. Ringer's lactate

Answer: b. Dextrose 5% is isotonic and is a good vehicle for potassium. 0.45% NaCl is hypotonic as is dextrose in 0.45%. Ringer's lactate contains components that mimic the concentration of electrolytes in blood.

7. The nurse gives a heparin injection with a tuberculin syringe that has what volume?

Answer:_____1 ml_____

8. The nurse gives Demerol IM to an adult by choosing which sized needle?
   a. 16 gauge
   b. 18 gauge
   c. 23 gauge
   d. 26 gauge

Answer: c. a 21-23 gauge needle is appropriate for an IM injection.

9. The nurse is giving a unit of packed RBCs. Which should the nurse look for if the client is having an acute hemolytic reaction? Select all that apply.
   a. Tachycardia
   b. Headache
   c. Fever
   d. Hypertension
   e. Dyspnea
   f. Back pain

Answer: a. b. e. f. Clinical manifestations of an acute hemolytic reaction are tachycardia, headache, dyspnea, and back pain.

10. The nurse should use what gauge of needle to administer blood?

Answer: _____16 gauge_____

11. When giving IV therapy to a client, it would be necessary for the nurse to include which of the following aspects of the procedure?
    a. Make a time strip on the bag with a felt tip marker.
    b. Change the tubing every 24 hours.
    c. Replace the IV solution with the same solution when the current bag runs out.
    d. Avoid letting an IV bag hang more than 24 hours

Answer: d. The IV bag cannot be kept hanging for more than 24-72 hours. Don't replace the bag with the same bag because the order could have changed. Don't use a felt tipped marker on the IV bag because it can leach through the plastic and contaminate the solution.

12. The nurse should include the following when administering an IV solution?
    a. Choose a microdrip chamber for medications given to a child.
    b. Set the end time of an infusion pump to give off an alarm 20 minutes before the scheduled end time.
    c. Select a macrodrip chamber for medications given to a geriatric client.
    d. Choose a volume-controlled administration set to deliver a large amount of IV solution.

Answer: a. A microdrip chamber should be used for both children and geriatric clients. A volume-controlled administration set delivers a small amount of IV solution. The alarm should go off when 50 cc of solution are remaining in the bag.

13. The nurse hangs which of the following for a client with thrombocytopenia?
    a. Whole blood
    b. Packed RBCs
    c. Platelets
    d. Albumin

Answer: c. A client with thrombocytopenia needs platelets.

14. A nurse cares for a client with a peripheral IV. Which would indicate the client is experiencing hypervolemia? Select all that apply.
    a. Nausea and vomiting
    b. Headache
    c. Dyspnea
    d. Hypertension
    e. Fever
    f. Tachycardia

Answer: c. d. f. Clinical manifestations of hypervolemia with intravenous therapy include dyspnea, hypertension, tachycardia, coughing, pulmonary edema, cyanosis, rales, and increased venous pressure. Nausea, vomiting, and fever are clinical manifestations of a pyrogenic reaction.

15. The nurse is caring for a client with an IV that is experiencing dyspnea, hypotension, a weak and rapid pulse, a decreased level of consciousness, and cyanosis. What is a priority nursing intervention?
    a. Notify the physician
    b. Place the client in a Trendelenburg position
    c. Give oxygen
    d. Stop the IV

Answer: d. The symptoms are classic of an air embolism so the IV should be stopped before giving O2, putting the client in a Trendelenburg position and notifying the physician.

16. The client is receiving fresh frozen plasma. The nurse should follow what lab results to see if the therapy is working?
    a. Hemoglobin and hematocrit
    b. Platelets
    c. Prothrombin time and partial thromboplastin time
    d. White blood cells

Answer: c. Fresh frozen plasma will improve the clotting of the client so the PT and PTT will improve. Hemoglobin/hematocrit are evaluated for giving pRBCs. The platelet count is measured when giving platelets and the WBC level will be measured when giving granulocytes.

17. You are teaching a class on controlled substances. What should you include as part of the class?
    a. There is no accepted medical use for a Schedule I controlled substance.
    b. Examples of Schedule II drugs include glutethimide, secobarbital, and hydrocodone.
    c. Schedule III controlled substances have a high potential for abuse.
    d. Schedule IV controlled substances are the same as an over-the-counter medication.

Answer: a. There is no accepted medical use for a Schedule I controlled substance. Glutethimide, secobarbital, and hydrocodone are schedule III drugs. Schedule II drugs have a high potential for abuse. Schedule IV drugs are not the same as over-the-counter medications.

18. Guaifenesin belongs to what class of controlled substances?
    a. Schedule II
    b. Schedule III
    c. Schedule IV
    d. Schedule V

Answer: d. Guaifenesin is a schedule V medication, with the lowest abuse potential.

19. The nurse is giving a client blood. Which of the following means that the nurse does not understand how to give blood?
    a. Run the blood slowly for the first 15 minutes at 20 drops per minute.
    b. Establish the required flow rate after 15 minutes if no signs of a reaction.
    c. Transfuse the blood slowly over six hours.
    d. Assess the vitals every 30 minutes until 1 hour after the transfusion.

Answer: c. Blood should be transfused over four hours. The rest of the choices are correct.

20. Which of the following clients is most appropriate to receive a central venous catheter?
    a. A dehydrated client with hypokalemia who needs fluid and electrolyte replacement.
    b. A client with cancer of the esophagus who is receiving chemotherapy.
    c. A client with an infection who needs short-term antibiotics.
    d. A client who is postoperative and is experiencing nausea after surgery.

Answer: b. A client with cancer needs a central venous catheter because it causes less irritation to the veins when giving chemotherapy. The other clients do not need this form of long term IV therapy.

21. The nurse should question the use of which drug for use in a client with glaucoma?
    a. Diamox
    b. Pilocarpine
    c. Atropine Sulfate
    d. Mannitol

Answer: c. Atropine is used to dilate the eyes but can precipitate an attack of glaucoma.

22. The nurse is giving a beta blocker to a client with glaucoma. What would indicate that there is a serious adverse reaction?
    a. Photophobia
    b. Blurry vision
    c. Drop in blood pressure
    d. Worsening of asthma

Answer: d. All of these are adverse reactions to beta blockers; however, the most serious adverse reaction is a worsening of the client's asthma.

23. What does a nurse give to a client with keratitis?
    a. Acyclovir
    b. Diamox
    c. Scopolamine
    d. Stoxil

Answer: d. Stoxil is used to treat inflammation of the cornea such as is seen in keratitis. Scopolamine dilates the eyes, acyclovir is used for Herpes zoster of the eyes and Diamox is used for glaucoma.

24. The nurse is administering Timoptic in each eye. Which comment does the client say indicating the need for more teaching?
    a. "I must wash my hands before putting in the drops."
    b. "This drug will decrease the fluid in my eye."
    c. "I need to take this until my eye pressure is normal."
    d. "Adverse reactions include dizziness and double vision."

Answer: c. Timoptic is used for glaucoma and should be taken for the duration of the person's life. Adverse reactions include dizziness and double vision.

25. The nurse tells client that the best position for instilling nose spray is to what?
    a. Bend the head forward
    b. Push the nare to the side
    c. Tilt the head backward
    d. Open the mouth to facilitate breathing

Answer: c. Tilting the head back helps get the nose spray into the nostrils.

26. You are assigned to give eyedrops to a client getting ready for cataract surgery. What kind of eye drop are you to give?
    a. An osmotic diuretic
    b. A miotic agent
    c. A mydriatic agent
    d. A thiazide diuretic

Answer: c. A mydriatic agent dilates the pupils, which is necessary before surgery. The other medications are not indicated in cataract surgery.

27. The nurse is giving a topical anti-infective whenever she gives the following: Select all that apply.
    a. Amoxicillin
    b. Polymixin B
    c. Neomycin
    d. Ceclor
    e. Chloramphenicol
    f. Biaxin

Answer: b. c. e. Polymixin B, Neomycin, and Chloramphenicol are examples of topical anti-infectives. The others are oral antibiotic agents.

28. A client has Meniere's disease and asks why Antivert is being prescribed. How does the nurse respond?
    a. It will control the vertigo.
    b. It will help you sleep.
    c. It will decrease your pain.
    d. It will control your nausea.

Answer: d. Antivert is a medication that controls nausea caused by severe vertigo but doesn't directly affect the vertigo.

29. A client is receiving phenylephrine (Neo-Synephrine). What should the nurse monitor the client for? Select all that apply.
    a. Urinary retention
    b. Dry skin
    c. Hypertension
    d. Tachycardia
    e. Headache
    f. Decreased sensitivity to light

Answer: c. d. e. Side effects of Neo-Synephrine include hypertension, headache, and tachycardia.

30. The nurse is taking a medication history from a client with herpes simplex of the eye. The nurse should ask if the client is taking which of the following drugs?
    a. Viroptic
    b. Cromolyn
    c. Stoxil
    d. Diamox

Answer: a. Viroptic is an anti-viral agent used to treat viral infections of the eye, such as herpes simplex.

31. The nurse understands that a client is to get which of the following drugs to paralyze the ciliary body muscles?
    a. Phenylephrine
    b. Homatropine
    c. Paredrine
    d. Cromolyn

Answer: b. Homatropine is a cycloplegic mydriatic that paralyzes the ciliary body muscles.

32. A client has been receiving IV theophylline and the doctor discontinues the medication to begin an immediate-release form of the medication. When should the first dose of the oral medication be given?
    e. Right after stopping the IV theophylline
    f. Begin 4-6 hours after stopping the IV theophylline
    g. Begin the oral dose at bedtime
    h. Start the oral dose with morning medications

Answer: b. The dose should be given 4-6 hours after stopping the IV theophylline. Giving it right away risks theophylline toxicity. The half-life of theophylline is 3-15 hours.

33. The client with acute asthma has inspiratory and expiratory wheezing along with a decreased FEV. What class of prescribed drugs should be given first to the client?
    a. Oral steroids
    b. Bronchodilators
    c. Inhaled steroids
    d. Mucolytics

Answer: b. The client is in an immediate need for a bronchodilator. Steroids are too slow-acting and mucolytics are unnecessary in asthma as there is very little mucus production.

34. The nurse is treating a client with asthma who is to be on theophylline. Which is an appropriate question to ask the client?
    a. Are you a diabetic on insulin?
    b. Do you take Tagamet?
    c. Do you regularly take aspirin?
    d. Do you exercise routinely?

Answer: b. Tagamet can reduce theophylline clearance and can increase the amount of the drug in the system, necessitating dosage adjustments. The other drugs have no effect on theophylline.

35. After teaching a client to use a beclomethasone inhaler, what does the client say to indicate that the teaching has been successful?
    a. I will limit myself to 2 cups of coffee per day.
    b. I will take it with meals to mask the taste.
    c. I will take it before bedtime every night.
    d. I will rinse my mouth after each use.

Answer: d. Oral steroid inhalers can cause oral Candidiasis so the mouth should be washed out after using the inhaler.

36. The client is being instructed as to how to use cromolyn sodium. Which indicates the client needs further instruction?
    a. If I don't feel better in 2-3 weeks, I will stop taking the medication.
    b. I will call the doctor if I get severe coughing from the drug.
    c. I have to take the medication even when I feel good.
    d. I do not need to stop my other medications just because I am taking this one.

Answer: a. The drug may take 4-8 weeks to take effect. It can be taken with other medications for asthma and must be taken even when feeling well. It cannot be abruptly stopped or it could trigger an asthma attack.

37. The client is being instructed on how to use a metered dose inhaler. What should the nurse tell the patient to do?
    a. Hold the breath for three seconds after using the inhaler
    b. Take a quick breath when activating the canister
    c. Activate the canister at the beginning of a slow deep breath
    d. Place the canister six inches in front of an open mouth

Answer: c. The canister should be in the mouth or a maximum of 2 inches in front of the mouth. A fast breath is not indicated. It should be activated at the beginning of a slow deep breath with holding of the breath for at least 5 seconds after the medication is administered.

38. What are the appropriate inhalation drugs for inflammation? Select all that apply.
    a. Cortisone
    b. Beclomethasone
    c. Dexamethasone
    d. Flunisolide (Aero-Bid)
    e. Prednisone
    f. Azmacort

Answer: b. d. f. Beclomethasone, Aero-Bid, and Azmacort are all inhaled steroids used for inflammation. The others are not inhaled medications.

39. The client with asthma asks why corticosteroids are best given by inhalation. What do you say?
    a. Inhaled medications are easier to take.
    b. The systemic adverse reactions are reduced.
    c. No weaning is required when stopping the drug.
    d. Oral care is not required.

Answer: b. Inhaled corticosteroids have fewer systemic effects. They must be tapered off and oral care is required to prevent Candidiasis.

40. The client has a sudden asthma attack. Which inhaler should the nurse give first?
    a. Albuterol
    b. Azmacort
    c. Flovent
    d. Cromolyn

Answer: a. Albuterol is an acute bronchodilator and should be given first. Azmacort and Flovent are steroids and can be given second. Cromolyn does not treat acute asthma attacks.

41. A client has pneumonia and is on a ventilator for respiratory distress. The chest x-ray shows left lower lob consolidation. The doctor orders respiratory treatments with Mucomyst. The nurse should monitor the client for what effects of the treatment?
    a. Bronchodilation
    b. Increased sputum
    c. Decreased level of consciousness
    d. Hypotension

Answer: b. Mucomyst is a mucolytic that will thin secretions so they are cleared better. Side effects include bronchospasm. It has no effect on level of consciousness or vital signs.

42. The nurse is caring for a client with an intractable cough. Which drug should be administered to the client?
    a. Rifampin
    b. Mucomyst
    c. Flovent
    d. Codeine

Answer: d. Codeine is a good cough suppressant that will decrease the cough. The others will have no effect on cough.

43. What should the nurse give as a priority to a client with a positive TB skin test but no evidence of active disease?
    a. Repeat skin test in 6 months.
    b. Isoniazid for 12 months.
    c. Multidrug therapy for at least 12 months.
    d. Streptomycin for 12 months.

Answer: b. A client with a positive TB skin test needs isoniazid for 12 months. Multidrug therapy is reserved for those with active disease. Skin tests will be positive in any repeat test.

44. The nurse is giving a client isoniazid. How should the medication be given to absorb the best?
    a. On an empty stomach
    b. With antacids to relieve upset stomach
    c. With food
    d. Thirty minutes after meals.

Answer: a. Isoniazid should be given one hour before meals or two hours after meals for better absorption. It should not be given with antacids.

45. You are caring for a client with COPD and pneumonia. After removing the endotracheal tube, which order should be in question?
    a. Continuation of antibiotics.
    b. O2 per nasal cannula at 6 liters/minute
    c. Out of bed with assistance
    d. Continue nebulizer treatments

Answer: b. Giving oxygen at such high levels can reduce the respiratory drive to breathe in a client with COPD and can precipitate respiratory arrest.

46. Humidification is necessary for oxygen flow rates of greater than what for drying of the mucus membranes?
    a. 1 liter/min
    b. 2 liter/min
    c. 3 liter/min
    d. 4 liter/min

Answer: b. Humidification should be used for oxygen flow rates of 2 liters/minute or greater to prevent drying of the mucus membranes.

47. You are teaching a client on the appropriate use of nebulizers and metered dose inhalers. What should you include as part of your instructions?
    a. Metered dose inhalers require a gas flow rate of 6-10 liters/min
    b. Nebulizers give medication through a face mask or mouthpiece
    c. Nebulizers deliver medications in puffs
    d. Metered dose inhalers need to be refrigerated

Answer: b. Nebulizers give medication through a face mask or mouthpiece at a rate of 6-10 liters per minute. Metered dose inhalers give medications in puffs and generally do not need to be refrigerated.

48. Which of the following are adverse drug reactions for bronchodilators? Select all that apply.
    a. Headache
    b. Tachycardia
    c. Sneezing
    d. Back pain
    e. Palpitations
    f. Depression

Answer: a. b. e. Common adverse reactions for bronchodilators include headache, tachycardia and palpitations.

49. You are delegating nursing tasks. What task should you designate to the LPN?
    a. Monitor the client using a decongestant for drug effectiveness.
    b. Develop a teaching plan for effective coughing techniques for a client on an expectorant.
    c. Increase the O2 flow rate for a client receiving O2 by face mask.
    d. Give a nasal spray to a client with rhinitis.

Answer: d. The LPN can give a nasal spray. The registered nurse must develop teaching plans and monitor medication effectiveness. A doctor's order is required to increase the O2 flow rate.

50. A client is in status asthmaticus. What is a priority nursing action?
    a. Administer aminophylline IV per doctor's order.
    b. Monitor the respiratory status for signs of hypoxia.
    c. Give inhaled bronchodilator therapy as ordered.
    d. Provide emotional support.

Answer: c. While all are appropriate actions, inhaled bronchodilators work the fastest and should be given first.

51. Which of the following is a priority activity for a nurse to do before administering digoxin?
    a. Assess the apical pulse for one minute.
    b. Palpate the radial pulse for 60 seconds.
    c. Monitor renal function tests.
    d. Assess the serum potassium.

Answer: a. The nurse should check the apical pulse for one minute before administering digoxin because a pulse less than 60 could mean digoxin toxicity. Renal function tests and serum potassium are important in giving digoxin but are not the priority action.

52. A client is in cardiac arrest. Which drug should the nurse give first?
    a. Atropine
    b. Epinephrine
    c. Lidocaine
    d. Atenolol

Answer: b. Epinephrine should be given first in anyone in cardiac arrest.

53. After teaching a client about atenolol, which indicates the diabetic client understands the instructions given?
    a. It may cause hyperglycemia.
    b. It may mask an early indication of hypoglycemia.
    c. It may increase the action of insulin.
    d. It may lessen the effectiveness of insulin.

Answer: b. Atenolol is a beta-blocker that depresses heart rate and prevents tachycardia, one of the first signs of hypoglycemia.

54. The nurse is taking care of a client with hypertension. Which drug should be administered?
    a. Mexiletine
    b. Dyazide
    c. Digoxin
    d. Warfarin

Answer: b. Dyazide is a medication given for hypertension. Digoxin is given for congestive heart failure. Mexiletine is an antiarrhythmic and warfarin is a blood thinner.

55. The client is receiving nitroglycerin for angina. What is the action of nitroglycerin on the body?
    a. Increase afterload
    b. Increase preload
    c. Constrict the arteries
    d. Dilate the veins

Answer: d. Nitroglycerin dilates the veins which decreases the preload to the heart, thus decreasing the workload on the heart.

56. The nurse is caring for a client with atrial fibrillation. Which drug concentration will double if given with quinidine?
    a. Lasix
    b. Digoxin
    c. Propranolol
    d. Dyazide

Answer: b. The giving of digoxin and quinidine together has the potential to double the concentration of the digoxin.

57. The nurse is giving amiodarone in order to treat which kind of arrhythmia?
    a. Sinus bradycardia
    b. Bundle branch block
    c. Ventricular arrhythmia
    d. Junctional rhythm

Answer: c. Amiodarone is an anti-arrhythmic used in the treatment of life-threatening ventricular arrhythmias.

58. Which is a priority nursing intervention for a client receiving adenosine for SVT?
    a. Document the presence of peripheral pulses.
    b. Monitor the pulse oximetry
    c. Assure the IV is in the antecubital vein.
    d. Prepare for emergency defibrillation.

Answer: c. Adenosine must be given in a large vein close to the heart because of its short half-life. This is the priority nursing intervention although the other choices are appropriate.

59. A client on Viagra is also experiencing angina for which the doctor has prescribed nitroglycerin as needed. What should the nurse tell the client about the taking of these two medications?
    a. Viagra should not be used within 24 hours of taking nitroglycerin.
    b. Nitroglycerin and Viagra should be taken at the same time.
    c. Viagra is not effective when used with nitroglycerin.
    d. The effect of nitroglycerin is impaired when used with Viagra.

Answer: a. Viagra and nitroglycerin together can cause severe hypotension so Viagra should not be used within 24 hours of taking nitroglycerin.

60. Which adverse reaction should the nurse assess in an elderly client receiving a continuous infusion of lidocaine?
    a. Hypertension
    b. Osteoarthritis
    c. Confusion
    d. Decreased visual acuity

Answer: c. Lidocaine is an antiarrhythmic used for ventricular arrhythmias. It can cause confusion in elderly adults.

61. The nurse is giving a beta blocker for unstable angina because it has which of the following actions?
    a. It increases myocardial contractility
    b. It decreases heart rate
    c. To promote a cardiovascular fluid shift
    d. For coronary artery vasodilation

Answer: b. Beta blockers decrease the heart rate, lessening the workload of the heart.

62. What is a priority nursing action when giving a client an ACE inhibitor?
    a. Monitor the blood pressure closely for 2 hours after the first dose.
    b. Begin with a high dose and then taper down the dose.
    c. Give potassium supplements to the client.
    d. Begin with daily dosing followed by every other day dosing.

Answer: a. ACE inhibitors can have first dose hypotension so the client must be monitored closely for two hours after the first dose.

63. The nurse is instructing a client on the use of Plavix. Which client statement indicates an understanding of the use of the drug?
    a. "I should ambulate slowly."
    b. "I may experience hypotension."
    c. "I should use caution taking other drugs that cause bleeding."
    d. "I should take a stool softener while on this drug."

Answer: c. Plavix is a blood thinner that should be taken with caution when taking other drugs that cause bleeding. It can cause hypertension and diarrhea as well.

64. The nurse should monitor a client with a heart attack that is receiving IV streptokinase for what serious adverse reaction?
    a. Intracranial hemorrhage
    b. Intractable nausea
    c. Extension of myocardial infarction
    d. Pulmonary embolism

Answer: a. Streptokinase thins the blood, putting the client at risk for intracranial hemorrhage or other hemorrhaging event.

65. The nurse is caring for a client on Lipitor. The client drinks 6-12 beers per day. What should the nurse look out for as a potentially serious adverse reaction to the drug?
    a. Nephrotoxicity
    b. Hypertension
    c. Hepatotoxicity
    d. Dyspepsia

Answer: c. Both alcohol and Lipitor rely on the liver for metabolism so that taking both can cause hepatotoxicity.

66. The client understands that the Zantac he is taking does what?
    a. Decreases gastric acid levels
    b. Changes hormonal levels.
    c. Increases pepsin levels
    d. Decreases pH levels.

Answer: a. Zantac is an H2-blocker that decreases levels of gastric acid in the stomach.

67. Which of the following should the nurse tell the client who is taking Carafate?
    a. It reduces gastric acid production
    b. It is to be given at breakfast time.
    c. Separate the taking of Carafate with other drugs by 2 hours.
    d. Carafate acts against H. pylori.

Answer: c. Carafate can't be taken within 2 hours of other drugs because it can bind with the other drugs, decreasing their absorption.

68. Which is a priority drug to give to a client who has gastroesophageal reflux disease (GERD)?
    a. Cytoprotectors
    b. Antibiotics
    c. Proton pump inhibitors
    d. Anticholinergics

Answer: c. Proton pump inhibitors are a first line treatment in the treatment of GERD.

69. The nurse should assess which of the following body systems while giving IV Tagamet to the client?
    a. Urinary system
    b. Immune system
    c. Respiratory system
    d. Cardiovascular system

Answer: d. IV Tagamet can cause dysrhythmias and hypotension so the cardiovascular system should be monitored.

70. The nurse should monitor the client taking Prevacid for which adverse reactions? Select all that apply.
    a. Headache
    b. Oliguria
    c. Anxiety
    d. Dry mouth
    e. Diarrhea
    f. Decreased appetite

Answer: a. d. e. Prevacid is a proton pump inhibitor which can have the adverse reactions of headache, dry mouth, and diarrhea.

71. The client is experiencing peptic ulcer disease due to
    H. pylori. Which drug combinations should be given?
    Biaxin is given along with what?
    a. Tetracycline and sodium bicarbonate
    b. Flagyl and Amphogel
    c. Amoxicillin and Prilosec
    d. Penicillin and Axid

Answer: c. Biaxin is given along with amoxicillin and Prilosec
for the treatment of H. pylori infections.

72. The nurse tells the client that which antacid has the
    side effect of constipation?
    a. Magaldrate (Riopan)
    b. Maalox
    c. Aluminum carbonate (Basaljel)
    d. Milk of Magnesia

Answer: c. All aluminum-containing antacids have the side
effect of constipation.

73. The nurse is caring for a client with a 15 year history of gastric ulcers. What should be taken by the client for minor aches and pains?
    a. Acetaminophen
    b. Buffered aspirin
    c. Plain aspirin
    d. Ibuprofen

Answer: a. Acetaminophen is the only analgesic listed that doesn't exacerbate gastric ulcers.

74. Which of the following antacids should the nurse question giving to the client with gastric ulcer and CHF?
    a. Magaldrate (Riopan)
    b. TUMS
    c. Milk of Magnesia
    d. Sodium bicarbonate

Answer: d. Sodium bicarbonate contains a lot of sodium, which is contraindicated in large doses in clients who have congestive heart failure.

75. The nurse is providing a medication schedule for a client taking Mylanta for gastritis. To promote best absorption, this drug should be given when? Select all that apply.
    a. At bedtime
    b. 1 hour before meals
    c. Immediately after meals
    d. Upon arising in the morning
    e. 1 hour after meals
    f. Thirty minutes after meals

Answer: a. b. e. Mylanta can be given one hour before meals, one hour after meals or at bedtime. It should not be given first thing in the morning.

76. A client giving a medication history tells you she is in the early stages of pregnancy. Which drug should be immediately discontinued?
    a. Misoprostol (Cytotec)
    b. Docusate
    c. Magnesium Hydroxide
    d. Pepto-Bismol

Answer: a. Cytotec is a medication that can cause inadvertent miscarriages and should be discontinued in early pregnancy.

77. The nurse is giving a client Tagamet. Which of the following adverse reactions should be watched out for? Select all that apply.
   a. Tinnitus
   b. Alopecia
   c. Diarrhea
   d. Mental confusion
   e. Dizziness
   f. Dyspepsia

Answer: c. d. e. Tagamet has the potential to cause diarrhea, mental confusion, and dizziness, especially in the elderly.

78. The nurse chooses the best antacid for the client because of which characteristic?
   a. Sweet-tasting, cathartic and effective for a long period of time.
   b. Short acting and readily absorbed
   c. Not absorbed by the body and acts as a laxative
   d. Decreases acidity without constipation or diarrhea.

Answer: d. The ideal antacid decreases acidity without constipation or diarrhea.

79. After giving Actigall with a client who has gallbladder disease, the nurse expects the priority outcome to be what?
    a. Decreased vomiting
    b. Increased comfort
    c. Decreased stone formation
    d. Decreased bile production

Answer: c. Actigall acts on the gallbladder to decrease stone formation. The patient will not have any immediate improvement in symptoms.

80. The nurse has given Compazine several times to a client experiencing vomiting. Which adverse reactions should the nurse be looking out for?
    a. Bradycardia
    b. Weight loss
    c. Akathisia
    d. Orthostatic hypotension
    e. Acute dystonia
    f. Oliguria

Answer: c. d. e. Compazine is a phenothiazine-type antiemetic that can cause extrapyramidal symptoms such s dystonia and akathisia. It can also cause orthostatic hypotension.

81. The client is receiving somatropin (Humatrope). What should the nurse tell the client to do?
    a. Get an annual bone age assessment.
    b. Schedule a fasting blood sugar annually if there is a family history of diabetes mellitus.
    c. Record height weekly and report linear growth of 7-15 cm in the first year.
    d. Notify the physician if the urine output increases.
    e.

Answer: a. Somatropin is growth hormone. The client should get an annual bone age assessment to see if the epiphyseal plates have closed. Diabetes mellitus is likely to happen so fasting blood sugars are assessed more often than once per year. The growth in height with somatropin is normal.

82. Which of the following is an anticipated outcome for a client with diabetes insipidus receiving vasopressin injections?
    a. Urine output of 2500 cc/day
    b. Weight loss of 4 pounds in a week.
    c. Urine specific gravity of 1.005
    d. Oral intake of 4500 cc/day

Answer: a. With vasopressin injection, there should be less polyuria and polydipsia. The urine output of 2500 cc/day is normal. If the urine specific gravity is 1.005 and the oral intake is 4500 cc/day, the diabetes insipidus is not being treated adequately.

83. The client on vasopressin asks why they should avoid alcohol while on this medication. What do you say?
    a. Alcohol will increase vasoconstriction.
    b. Alcohol will decrease the antidiuretic effect.
    c. Alcohol will interfere with the absorption of vasopressin in the stomach.
    d. Alcohol will promote a hypersensitivity to vasopressin.

Answer: b. Alcohol actually causes vasodilatation. It decreases the antidiuretic effect of vasopressin.

84. The nurse recognizes that one of the following drugs is a first generation sulfonylurea in the treatment of diabetes? Select all that apply.
    a. Glipizide (Glucotrol)
    b. Tolbutamide (Orinase)
    c. Acarbose (Precose)
    d. Tolazamide (Tolinase)
    e. Chlorpropamide (Diabenese)
    f. Rosiglitazone (Avandia)

Answer: b. d. e. Orinase, Tolinase, and Diabenese are all first generation sulfonylurea medications. Precose and Avandia are not sulfonylurea medications and Glucotrol is a second generation sulfonylurea.

85. Before discharge, the nurse instructs a client on Cytomel to notify the physician if which of the following occurs?
    a. A pulse rate of 100 beats per minute.
    b. A weight loss of 5 pounds in two weeks.
    c. More frequent urination
    d. Excessive sleepiness
    e.

Answer: Cytomel is a drug used for hypothyroidism. If the pulse is too high, it may indicate the client is being over-medicated. Weight loss and diuresis are to be expected and sleepiness should resolve itself after the medication begins to work.

86. The best time to take Synthroid (levothyroxine) is when?
    a. One hour after a meal.
    b. With a bedtime snack.
    c. Thirty minutes before breakfast.
    d. Once a day with any meal.

Answer: c. Synthroid should be taken without food and so thirty minutes before breakfast is a good time to take the medication.

87. The nurse is giving the client Mestinon. The client should be monitored for which of the following adverse reactions?
    a. Constipation
    b. Decreased heart rate
    c. Hypertension
    d. Increased intraocular pressure.

Answer: b. Mestinon is used for the treatment of myasthenia gravis. The major side effects are decreased heart rate, diarrhea, and low blood pressure.

88. The nurse should monitor the client for which signs after giving Ativan IV to a client who has many seizures?
    a. Tachycardia
    b. Hypertension
    c. Tissue hypoxia
    d. Respiratory depression

Answer: d. Ativan can suppress the respiratory drive to breathe so the client needs to be monitored for signs of respiratory depression.

89. A client is taking Dilantin 200 mg daily. Which of the following is an adverse reaction that must be watched out for?
    a. Diarrhea
    b. Pruritus
    c. Sedation
    d. Hypertension

Answer: c. Dilantin is used for seizures. Side effects include sedation, constipation, and hypotension.

90. You are infusing Dilantin with which of the following solutions to control seizures?
    a. Normal saline
    b. D5W
    c. Lactated Ringer's solution
    d. D5W in 0.5 normal saline

Answer: a. Dilantin forms a precipitate with dextrose so it should only be infused with normal saline, which does not contain dextrose.

91. Dilantin is being given to a client for seizures. What should the nurse prepare to do?
    a. Maintain a level of between 30 and 50 micrograms per ml.
    b. Dilute the IV Dilantin with 5% dextrose
    c. Administer good oral hygiene.
    d. Give the medication intramuscularly.

Answer: c. Dilantin can cause gingival hyperplasia, which is treated with good oral hygiene. The normal therapeutic level is between 7.5 and 20 micrograms per ml. Dilantin should not be given intramuscularly or with dextrose.

92. The nurse should tell a client taking an oral retinoid to avoid which of the following items?
    a. Dairy products
    b. Carbonated beverages
    c. Extremely cold air
    d. Vitamin A supplements

Answer: d. An oral retinoid and vitamin A supplements, when taken together, can cause vitamin A toxicity.

93. The nurse is caring for a client who has been taking Accutane for the past two months. What is a priority condition that the nurse should report to the physician?
    a. Itching
    b. Depression
    c. Dry skin
    d. Headache

Answer: b. Accutane can cause all of these conditions but depression is the priority because it can lead to suicidal ideation in a client who is taking the drug.

94. The nurse is giving instructions to a client with itching to take an oral antihistamine to relieve itching. Which should be included in the instructions?
    a. The effects will be better if you take the medication around the clock.
    b. Take the medication only when the itching is at its worst.
    c. You can take the oral medication along with a topical antihistamine.
    d. Increase the dose of the oral antihistamine if the itching gets worse.

Answer: a. Antihistamines will work better if you take them around the clock. The sedation caused by these medications will diminished if it is taken this way.

95. A client has second-degree burns on the hands and arms. The client is being given Silvadene for topical antimicrobial effects. What instructions for taking the medication should be given?
    a. Wash the area with warm water before applying Silvadene.
    b. Apply a salve after the Silvadene to seal the medication into the burned area.
    c. Apply Silvadene using sterile technique
    d. Apply the medication only at bedtime.

Answer: a. The area should be washed with warm water before applying Silvadene. The medication does not need a salve to seal it and it doesn't have to be given using sterile technique. It is generally applied twice a day.

96. A 22-year old female has been diagnosed with acne and is starting on tetracycline. What is a priority question to ask the client before starting therapy?
    a. How long have you had acne?
    b. When was your last menstrual period?
    c. How many times a day do you wash your face?
    d. Have you been taking any oral medication for acne?

Answer: b. Tetracycline can cause birth defects so it is important that the client not be pregnant while taking it. She should use birth control while taking the medication.

97. The nurse tells the client that what is a good treatment for Raynaud's phenomenon?
    a. Nonsteroidal anti-inflammatory medication
    b. Corticosteroids
    c. Aspirin
    d. Calcium-channel blockers

Answer: d. Calcium channel blockers relieve vasospasm by dilating the vessels and can be used for attacks of Raynaud's phenomenon.

98. Allopurinol and colchicine have been prescribed for a client with gout and diabetes. How should you instruct the client?
    a. Tell them that blood glucose values may not be valid.
    b. Urine sugar tests may not be valid.
    c. Protein restrictions can lead to diabetic ketoacidosis.
    d. Protein cannot be restricted so you need to increase the dose of allopurinol.

Answer: b. Urine sugar tests may not be valid when taking these medications.

99. The nurse should give the following medications to a client with severe rheumatoid arthritis?
    a. Methotrexate
    b. Naproxen
    c. Aspirin
    d. Plaquenil

Answer: a. Methotrexate is reserved for clients with severe rheumatoid arthritis but monitoring for toxic effects is necessary.

100. Which of the following should a nurse consider before giving an opioid to a child?
    a. The child's age, weight, height, and respiratory status.
    b. Children are less susceptible to adverse reactions.
    c. Addiction is increased in children.
    d. Sedation is increased in children.

Answer: a. The child's age, weight, height and respiratory status must be assessed before giving a child an opioid. There is no evidence to suggest that there is increased sedation or addiction in children.

101.　　When giving a child Augmentin, the nurse should monitor the client for what?
a.　Constipation
b.　Polyuria
c.　Decreased temperature
d.　Increased bleeding

Answer: d. Augmentin is an anti-infective based on penicillin. Its side effects are increased bleeding times, diarrhea, and fever.

102.　　The nurse is instructing a class about antibiotics and UTIs. Which should be included in the class?
a.　E. coli is mostly resistant to penicillin medications.
b.　Sulfonamides are given for Pseudomonas infections
c.　Fluoroquinolones have limited use in the treatment of UTIs.
d.　Cephalosporins are the treatment of choice for those sensitive to penicillin.

Answer: a. E. coli is mostly resistant to penicillin medications. Sulfonamides do not work well against Pseudomonas. Fluoroquinolones are often used in the treatment of UTIs and Cephalosporins may have cross-reactivity to clients sensitive to penicillin.

103.   The nurse is admitting a client with suspected schizophrenia. Which of the following clinical manifestations should the nurse assess as a positive clinical manifestation of schizophrenia?
   a. Anhedonia and blunted affect.
   b. Hallucinations and delusional thinking
   c. Lack of motivation
   d. Abnormal movements of the mouth.

Answer: b. Both hallucinations and delusional thinking are positive manifestations of schizophrenia. Anhedonia and blunted affect are not positive manifestations of schizophrenia, nor is a lack of motivation. Abnormal movements of the mouth are side effects of taking medications for schizophrenia.

104.   The nurse is caring for an Alzheimer's patient who is taking Seroquel for paranoid ideations. Which adverse reactions should the nurse look out for?
   a. Hypertension
   b. Headache
   c. Bradycardia
   d. Diarrhea
   e. Dry mouth
   f. Tardive dyskinesia

Answer: b. e. f. Seroquel is an antipsychotic used for psychotic disorders. Adverse reactions include orthostatic hypotension, headache, tachycardia, constipation, dry mouth and tardive dyskinesia.

105.   What should the nurse tell a client who is on an antidepressant drug?
a. Drink low calorie beverages.
b. Instruct the client to take the drug on an empty stomach.
c. Tell the client that urinary frequency is a side effect of the drug.
d. The client should be monitored for bradycardia before giving the drug.

Answer: a. Antidepressants are used to treat depression. Weight gain is one of the side effects of the drug so the client should avoid taking in extra calories.

Conclusion

I hope you received a ton of value from this book. Remember, practice makes perfect so you will have to repeat these readings.

If you enjoyed this book, would you be kind enough to leave a review on Amazon? Your review can help others to see what kinds of helpful resources are out there!

Thank you and good luck on your medical endeavors!

- Chase Hassen

Nurse Superhero

Highly Recommended Books for Success

1. NCLEX: Cardiovascular System : 105 Nursing Practice and Rationales to Easily Crush the NCLEX!

2. NCLEX: Emergency Nursing : 105 Practice Questions and Rationales to Easily Crush the NCLEX!

3. Lab Values: 137 Values You Know to Easily Pass The NCLEX!

4. EKG Interpretation: 24 Hours or Less to Easily Pass the ECG Portion of the NCLEX!

5. Fluid and Electrolytes: 24 Hours or Less to Absolutely Crush the NCLEX Exam!

6. Nursing Careers: Easily Choose What Nursing Career Will Make Your 12 Hour Shift a Blast!

7. Night Shift: 10 Survival Tips for Nurses to Get Through The Night!

8. <u>NCLEX: Endocrine System : 105 Nursing Practice Questions and Rationales to EASILY Crush the NCLEX!</u>

And **MUCH MUCH MORE**! Visit my amazon author page to see more at http://amzn.to/1HCtfSy

75506761R00064

Made in the USA
San Bernardino, CA
30 April 2018